I0427145

MIND DIET COOKBOOK FOR SENIORS

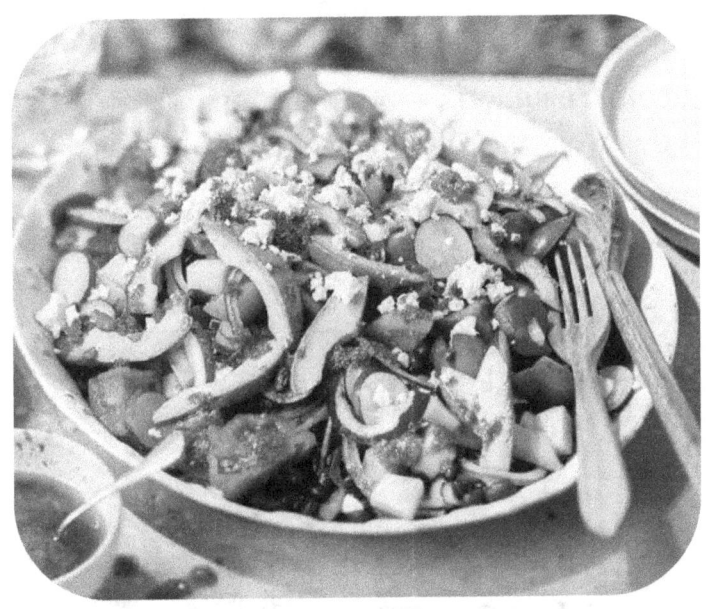

2000 DAYS OF TASTY, EASY AND DELICIOUS BRAIN BOOSTING RECIPES TO HELP FIGHT MEMORY DISORDERS, ALZHEIMER'S & DEMENTIA FOR HEALTHIER LIFE (WITH 98 DAYS MEAL PLAN)

CARLY EVELYN

(Copyright © 2024 Carly Evelyn)
All rights reserved. No part of this book may be reproduced, stored, or transmitted by any means—whether auditory, graphic, mechanical, or electronic—without written permission of both the copyright owner and the above publisher of this book. Unauthorized reproduction of any part of this work is illegal and is punishable by law.

SCAN TO GET MORE BOOKS BY THIS AUTHOR FOR A HEALTHIER LIFESTYLE

IF YOU ARE STUCK, WHILE PREPARING ANY RECIPES IN THIS COOKBOOK, YOU CAN REACH THE AUTHOR AT CARLYEVLCUISINEGUIDE@GMAIL.COM FOR GUIDANCE

TABLE OF CONTENTS

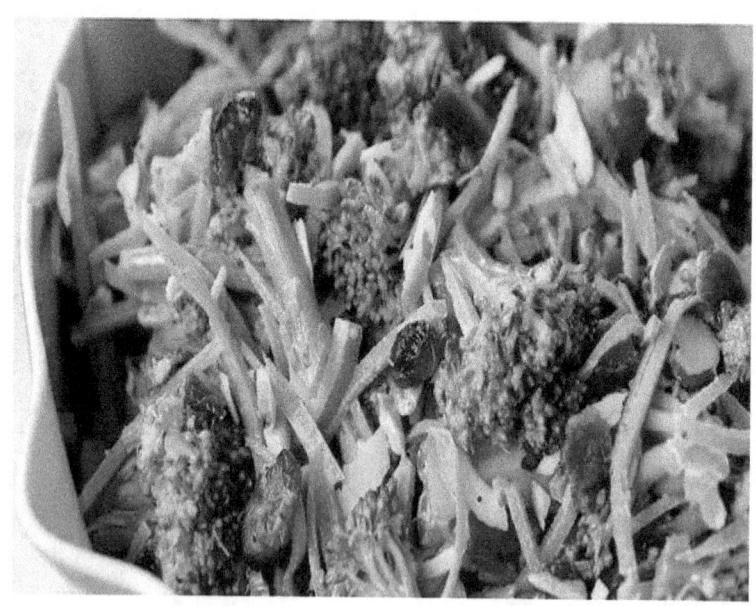

INTRODUCTION

In the bustling heart of the city, where skyscrapers touched the sky and the rhythm of life never seemed to slow, there lived an extraordinary couple, Robert and Evelyn. They had spent a lifetime together, navigating the bustling streets and creating a mosaic of memories. However, as the years advanced, a cruel twist of fate cast a shadow over their golden years. Both were grappling with the early stages of dementia, a relentless thief that stole the clarity from their minds.

Amidst the urban chaos, a beacon of hope emerged in the form of Dr. Harper, a renowned nutritionist who specialized in the impact of diet on cognitive health. Intrigued by the challenges faced by the elderly couple, Dr. Harper proposed a revolutionary dietary approach, rich in brain-boosting nutrients and anti-inflammatory foods.

Robert and Evelyn, armed with determination and a desire to reclaim their shared history, embraced the new diet with open hearts. The bustling city became their playground for sourcing the freshest produce, and their kitchen transformed into a laboratory of culinary experimentation.

Leafy greens, berries, nuts, and fatty fish became the staples of their daily meals. The city's diverse markets offered a rich tapestry of ingredients that not only tantalized their taste buds but also held the promise of cognitive rejuvenation. Their once mundane routine of fast food and convenience snacks gave way to a vibrant array of colors and flavors that mirrored the renewal happening within.

As the weeks went by, a subtle change began to unfold. The forgotten names and misplaced keys became less frequent. Robert's witty banter returned, and Evelyn's eyes sparkled with a renewed sense of recognition. Their apartment, once cluttered with sticky notes to jog their memories, now bore witness to a remarkable transformation.

Word of their journey spread through the city like wildfire. Dr. Harper's approach, once met with skepticism, gained credibility as Robert and Evelyn's story inspired others facing similar battles. Seniors across the city embarked on their own culinary odysseys, forging alliances with local farmers and exploring the cornucopia of healthful foods that the urban landscape had to offer.

The city, often accused of being indifferent, witnessed a collective effort to support its aging population. Community gardens sprouted in neighborhoods, providing a source of fresh produce for those determined to follow in Robert and Evelyn's footsteps. The urban rhythm seemed to harmonize with the beat of resilience and renewal.

In the heart of the city, Robert and Evelyn became living testaments to the power of a carefully curated diet in managing cognitive decline. Their story rippled through the streets, echoing a message of hope and transformation. The bustling metropolis, often accused of grinding down its inhabitants, had become an unexpected ally in the journey toward cognitive well-being for its cherished seniors.

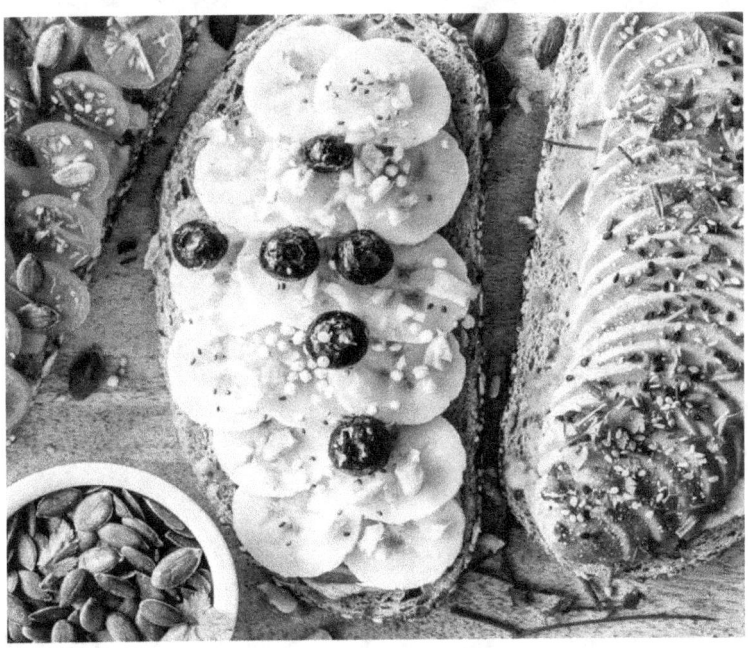

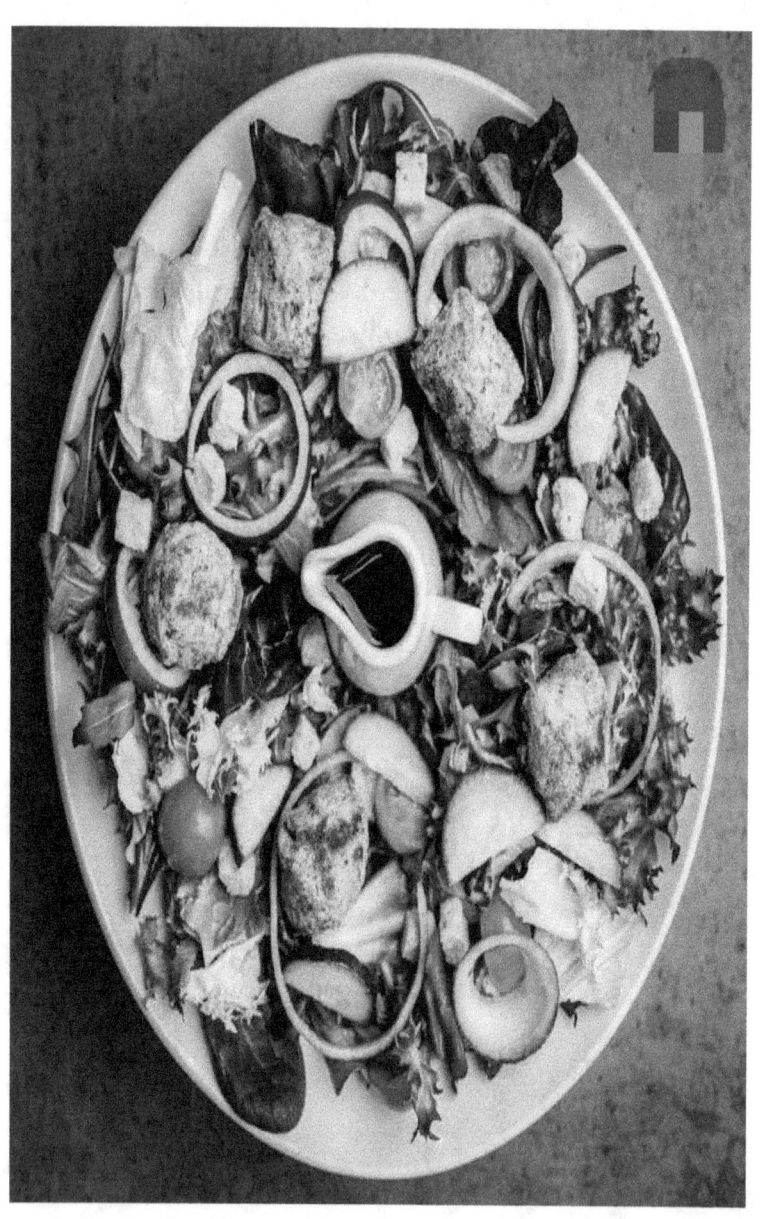

MAKING THE BRAIN DIET WORK FOR YOU

In the dynamic fabric of contemporary existence, where demands persist and diversions are plentiful, the concept of a "brain diet" has emerged as a source of optimism for those pursuing mental clarity and cognitive wellness. Achieving success with the brain diet entails more than merely altering your eating habits; it requires a comprehensive strategy that encompasses lifestyle, mindfulness, and a commitment to nurturing both the body and mind.

1. Embrace Nutrient-Rich Foods

- Commence by integrating brain-boosting foods into your daily meals. These encompass fatty fish abundant in omega-3 fatty acids (such as salmon and trout), antioxidant-rich berries (like blueberries and strawberries), nuts and seeds, leafy greens (such as spinach and kale), and whole grains.

- Explore a diverse array of vibrant fruits and vegetables to ensure a wide range of vitamins and minerals that bolster cognitive function.

2. Prioritize Healthy Fats

- Opt for beneficial fats found in avocados, olive oil, and nuts. These fats furnish essential nutrients for the brain, contributing to overall cognitive health.

3. Hydrate Your Brain

- Maintain adequate hydration. Dehydration can hinder concentration and cognitive function. Make water your primary beverage throughout the day.

4. Mindful Eating Practices

- Foster mindful eating habits by paying attention to the colors, textures, and flavors of your food. This not only enhances the pleasure of eating but also fosters a profound connection between your mind and body.

5. Reduce Processed Foods and Sugars

- Minimize consumption of processed foods and sugars, which can contribute to inflammation and negatively impact cognitive function. Opt for whole, unprocessed foods whenever feasible.

6. Include Brain-Boosting Herbs and Spices

- Experiment with herbs and spices known for their cognitive benefits. For instance, turmeric contains curcumin, renowned for its anti-inflammatory and antioxidant properties.

7. Plan Balanced Meals

- Design well-balanced meals incorporating a mix of carbohydrates, proteins, and healthy fats. This aids in maintaining stable blood sugar levels, ensuring a consistent supply of energy to the brain.

8. Incorporate Regular Physical Activity

- Engage in consistent physical activity. Exercise has been correlated with enhanced cognitive function and can amplify the efficacy of a brain-boosting diet.

9. Prioritize Sleep

- Ensure sufficient and quality sleep. Adequate sleep is pivotal for memory consolidation and overall brain health.

10. Cultivate Mental Well-Being

- Lastly, recognize the significance of mental well-being. Practice stress management techniques, involve yourself in activities that bring joy, and foster positive social connections.

Remain cognizant that tailoring the brain diet to suit your needs is not a one-size-fits-all endeavor. Pay heed to your body, exercise patience throughout the process, and be open to adjustments as necessary. Through dedication and a mindful approach, you can leverage the potential of nutrition to bolster cognitive health, leading to a more vibrant and gratifying life.

_____

_____

_____

_____

_____

_____

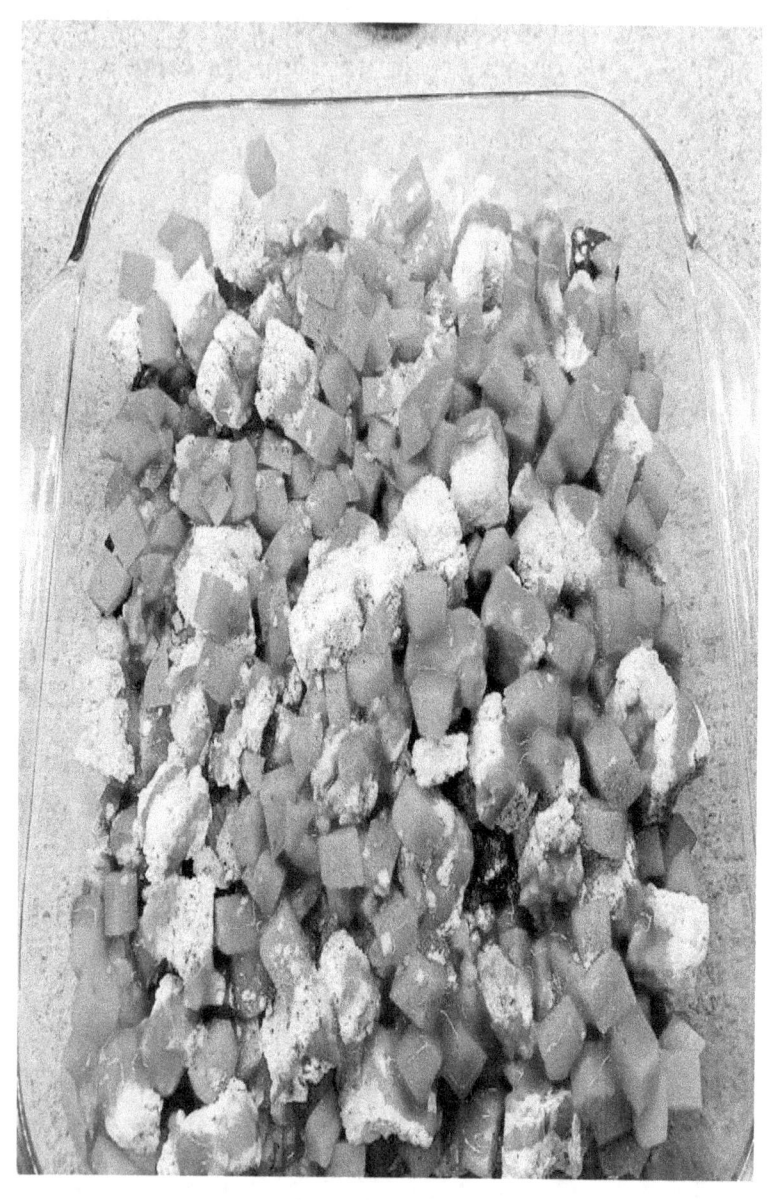

BREAKFAST RECIPES

Here are revamped versions of the recipes for each brain/mind diet dish, incorporating ingredients, preparation steps, measurement specifics, nutritional content, and approximate cooking durations—all provided in US units.

1. Banana-Almond Butter Overnight Oats

Ingredients
- 1/2 cup rolled oats
- 1/2 cup almond milk
- 1 ripe banana, mashed
- 1 tablespoon almond butter

Preparation
1. Combine rolled oats and almond milk in a jar.
2. Add mashed banana and almond butter.
3. Stir thoroughly, cover, and refrigerate overnight.
4. Give it a good stir in the morning and savor the deliciousness!

Nutritional Value
- Calories Around 350
- Protein 10g
- Fiber 8g
- Healthy Fats 15g

Cooking Time 5 minutes (plus overnight refrigeration)

2. High-Protein Veggie Egg Muffins

Ingredients
- 6 large eggs
- 1/2 cup diced bell peppers
- 1/2 cup diced tomatoes
- 1/4 cup diced onions
- Salt and pepper to taste
- 1/4 cup shredded cheese (optional)

Preparation
1. Preheat the oven to 350°F (175°C) and grease a muffin tin.
2. Beat eggs in a bowl, season with salt and pepper.
3. Mix in diced vegetables and cheese (if desired).
4. Pour the mixture into muffin cups and bake for 20-25 minutes until eggs are set.

Nutritional Value
- Calories Approximately 90 per muffin
- Protein 7g
- Healthy Fats 5g

Cooking Time 25 minutes

3. Greek Yogurt Berry Delight

Ingredients
- 1 cup Greek yogurt
- 1/2 cup mixed berries (blueberries, strawberries, raspberries)

Preparation
1. Spoon Greek yogurt into a bowl.
2. Top with a medley of mixed berries.

Nutritional Value
- Calories Approximately 200
- Protein 20g
- Fiber 5g

Cooking Time 5 minutes

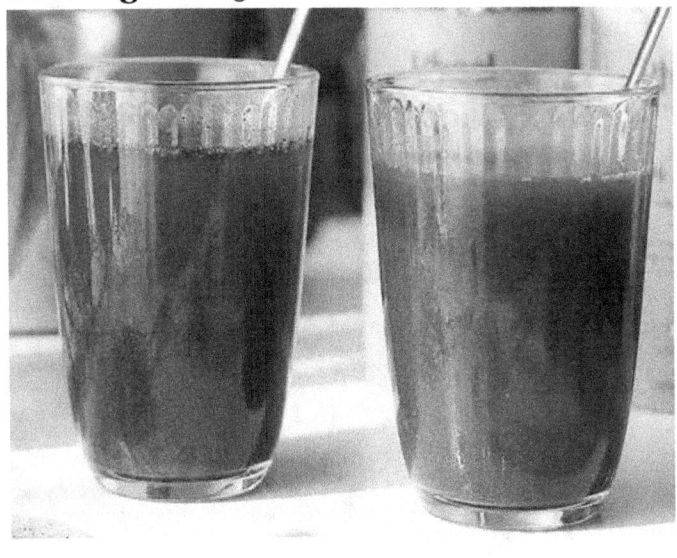

4. Whole-Grain Berry Pancakes

Ingredients

- 1 cup whole-grain pancake mix
- 3/4 cup water
- 1/2 cup mixed berries

Preparation

1. Blend pancake mix and water until smooth.
2. Cook pancakes on a griddle.
3. Crown them with an assortment of mixed berries.

Nutritional Value

- Calories Approximately 300
- Protein 8g
- Fiber 6g

Cooking Time 15 minutes

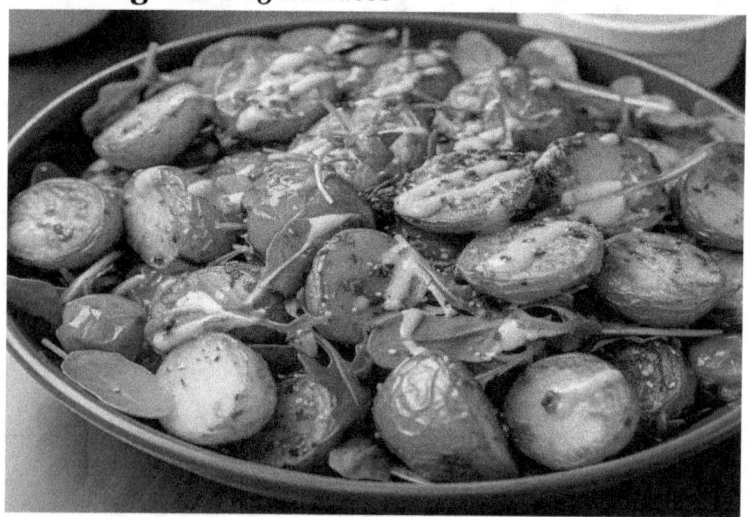

5. Nutty Fruit Oatmeal Powerhouse

Ingredients
- 1/2 cup rolled oats
- 1 cup water
- 2 tablespoons chopped nuts (almonds, walnuts)
- 1/2 cup diced fruit (apple, pear)

Preparation
1. Cook oats in water until achieving the desired consistency.
2. Garnish with chopped nuts and diced fruit.

Nutritional Value
- Calories Around 250
- Protein 7g
- Fiber 8g

Cooking Time 10 minutes

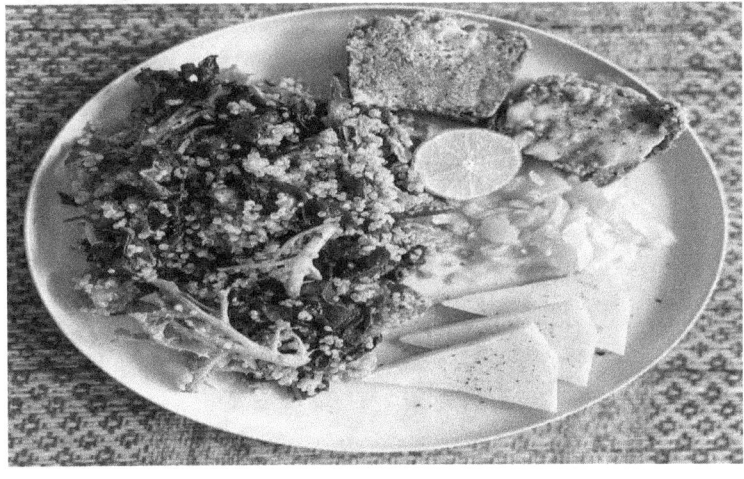

6. Avocado and Egg Harmony on Toast

Ingredients

- 1 slice whole-grain bread
- 1/2 avocado, mashed
- 1 egg, poached or fried
- Salt and pepper to taste

Preparation

1. Toast the whole-grain bread.
2. Spread mashed avocado on the toast.
3. Crown it with a poached or fried egg.
4. Season with salt and pepper.

Nutritional Value

- Calories Approximately 300
- Protein 10g
- Healthy Fats 15g

Cooking Time 10 minutes

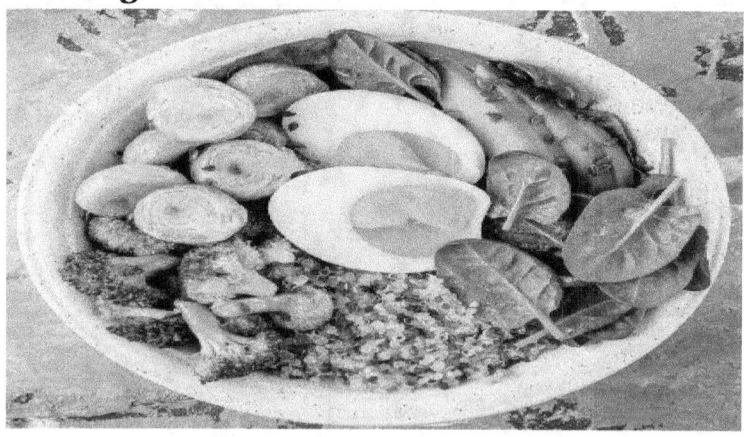

7. Chia-Coconut Smoothie Bowl

Ingredients
- 1 cup frozen mixed berries
- 1 banana
- 1/2 cup Greek yogurt
- 1 tablespoon chia seeds
- 1 tablespoon shredded coconut

Preparation
1. Blend frozen berries, banana, and Greek yogurt to create a smooth mixture.
2. Pour into a bowl and garnish with chia seeds and shredded coconut.

Nutritional Value
- Calories Approximately 300
- Protein 10g
- Fiber 12g

Cooking Time 5 minutes

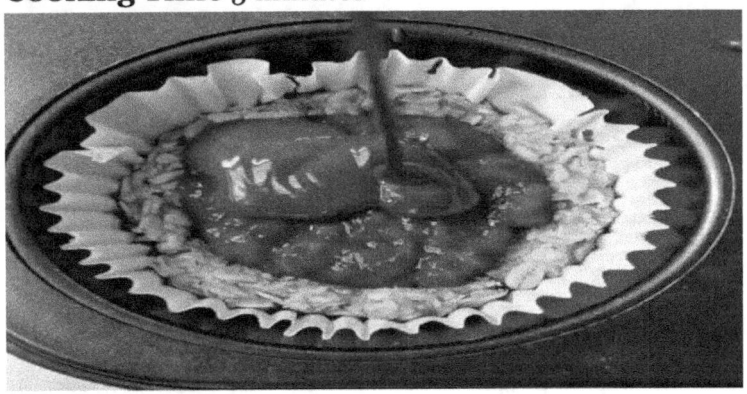

8. Savory Quinoa Bowl with Veggie Bliss and Soft-Boiled Egg

Ingredients

- 1/2 cup cooked quinoa
- Assorted veggies (bell peppers, spinach, cherry tomatoes)
- 1 soft-boiled egg
- Salt and pepper to taste

Preparation

1. Arrange cooked quinoa and assorted veggies in a bowl.
2. Crown it with a soft-boiled egg.
3. Season with salt and pepper.

Nutritional Value

- Calories Approximately 350
- Protein 15g
- Fiber 8g

Cooking Time 15 minutes

_____
_____
_____
_____
_____
_____
_____
_____

9. Whole-Grain Toast with Butter and Banana Bliss

Ingredients
- 1 slice whole-grain bread
- 1 tablespoon nut butter (almond or peanut)
- 1/2 banana, sliced

Preparation
1. Toast the whole-grain bread.
2. Spread nut butter on the toast.
3. Garnish with banana slices.

Nutritional Value
- Calories Approximately 250
- Protein 6g
- Healthy Fats 10g

Cooking Time 5 minutes

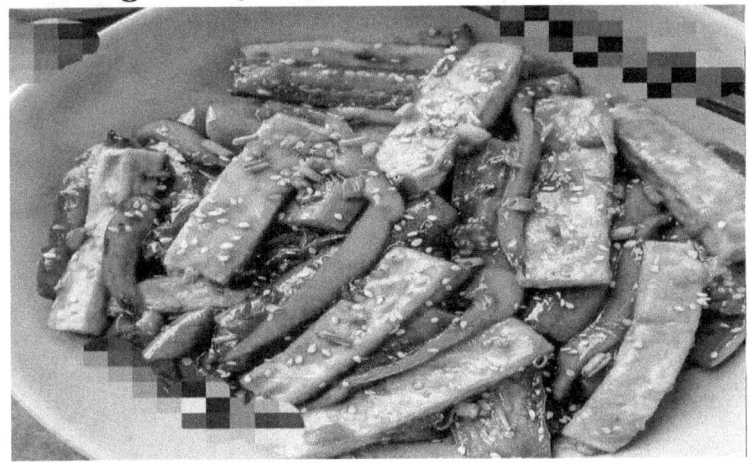

10. Vegetable Frittata with Cheese and Herbal Elegance

Ingredients

- 4 large eggs
- 1/2 cup diced bell peppers
- 1/4 cup diced onions
- 1/4 cup shredded cheese
- Fresh herbs (parsley, chives)
- Salt and pepper to taste

Preparation

1. Preheat the oven to 375°F (190°C).
2. Whisk eggs and combine with diced vegetables, cheese, and herbs.
3. Pour the mixture into a greased baking dish.
4. Bake for 20-25 minutes until the frittata is fully set.

Nutritional Value

- Calories Approximately 200
- Protein 12g
- Healthy Fats 15g

Cooking Time 25 minutes

LUNCH RECIPES

Here are comprehensive explanations of the recipes for mind-boosting dishes, providing details on ingredients, preparation methods, quantity measurements, nutritional values, and estimated cooking times—all presented in US units.

1. Greek Yogurt and Vegetables Power Bowl

Ingredients
- 1 cup Greek yogurt
- 1 cup mixed vegetables (cherry tomatoes, cucumbers, bell peppers)
- 1/4 cup crumbled feta cheese
- 1 tablespoon olive oil
- Salt and pepper to taste

Preparation
1. Place Greek yogurt in a bowl.
2. Add a mix of vegetables and crumbled feta on top.
3. Drizzle with olive oil and season with salt and pepper.

Nutritional Value
- Calories Approximately 350
- Protein 20g
- Fiber 5g

Cooking Time 5 minutes

2. Quinoa and Black Bean Salad

Ingredients
- 1 cup cooked quinoa
- 1/2 cup black beans, drained and rinsed
- 1/2 cup corn kernels
- 1/4 cup finely chopped red onion
- 1/4 cup chopped cilantro
- 2 tablespoons lime juice
- 1 tablespoon olive oil
- Salt and cumin to taste

Preparation
1. Combine quinoa, black beans, corn, red onion, and cilantro in a bowl.
2. Whisk together lime juice, olive oil, salt, and cumin in a separate bowl.
3. Pour the dressing over the quinoa mixture and toss.

Nutritional Value
- Calories Approximately 300
- Protein 10g
- Fiber 8g

Cooking Time 15 minutes

3. Mediterranean Chopped Salad

Ingredients
- 2 cups mixed greens
- 1/2 cup halved cherry tomatoes
- 1/4 cup diced cucumber
- 1/4 cup sliced Kalamata olives
- 1/4 cup crumbled feta cheese
- 2 tablespoons olive oil
- 1 tablespoon balsamic vinegar
- Salt and oregano to taste

Preparation
1. Combine mixed greens, cherry tomatoes, cucumber, olives, and feta in a large bowl.
2. Whisk together olive oil, balsamic vinegar, salt, and oregano in a small bowl.
3. Drizzle the dressing over the salad and toss gently.

Nutritional Value
- Calories Approximately 250
- Protein 8g
- Fiber 5g

Cooking Time 10 minutes

4. Egg and Avocado Sandwich

Ingredients

- 2 slices whole-grain bread
- 2 large eggs
- 1/2 avocado, sliced
- Salt and pepper to taste
- Optional hot sauce or salsa

Preparation

1. Toast the whole-grain bread slices.
2. Cook the eggs to your liking (fried, scrambled, or poached).
3. Layer avocado slices on one bread slice.
4. Place the cooked eggs on top and season with salt and pepper.
5. Top with the second bread slice. Add hot sauce or salsa if desired.

Nutritional Value

- Calories Approximately 350
- Protein 15g
- Healthy Fats 20g

Cooking Time 10 minutes

5. Turkey and Hummus Wrap

Ingredients
- 1 whole-grain wrap
- 4 ounces turkey breast slices
- 2 tablespoons hummus
- 1/2 cup mixed greens
- 1/4 cup julienned cucumber
- 1/4 cup shredded carrots

Preparation
1. Lay the whole-grain wrap on a flat surface.
2. Spread hummus over the wrap.
3. Layer turkey slices, mixed greens, cucumber, and shredded carrots.
4. Roll the wrap tightly, cut in half, and secure with toothpicks if needed.

Nutritional Value
- Calories Approximately 300
- Protein 20g
- Fiber 6g

Cooking Time 5 minutes

6. Zucchini and Ricotta Tostadas

Ingredients

- 2 small corn tortillas
- 1 medium zucchini, thinly sliced
- 1/2 cup ricotta cheese
- 1 tablespoon olive oil
- 1 clove garlic, minced
- Salt and pepper to taste
- Fresh basil for garnish

Preparation

1. Heat olive oil in a pan, add minced garlic, and sauté until fragrant.
2. Add zucchini slices and cook until tender. Season with salt and pepper.
3. In a separate pan, warm corn tortillas.
4. Spread ricotta cheese on each tortilla.
5. Top with sautéed zucchini and garnish with fresh basil.

Nutritional Value

- Calories Approximately 250
- Protein 10g
- Healthy Fats 15g

Cooking Time 15 minutes

7. Chicken Salad with Grapes and Almonds

Ingredients

- 1 cup cooked shredded chicken breast
- 1/2 cup halved red grapes
- 1/4 cup sliced almonds
- 1/4 cup diced celery
- 1/4 cup Greek yogurt
- 1 tablespoon mayonnaise
- Salt and pepper to taste
- Lettuce leaves for serving

Preparation

1. In a bowl, combine shredded chicken, grapes, almonds, celery, Greek yogurt, and mayonnaise.
2. Season with salt and pepper.
3. Serve the chicken salad in lettuce leaves.

Nutritional Value

- Calories Approximately 300
- Protein 25g
- Healthy Fats 15g

Cooking Time 10 minutes

8. Salmon and Quinoa Bowl

Ingredients

- 4 ounces salmon fillet
- 1/2 cup cooked quinoa
- 1 cup mixed vegetables (broccoli, carrots, bell peppers)
- 1 tablespoon olive oil
- Lemon wedges for serving
- Salt and pepper to taste

Preparation

1. Season the salmon with salt and pepper.
2. In a pan, heat olive oil and cook the salmon until flaky.
3. In a bowl, assemble cooked quinoa and mixed vegetables.
4. Place the cooked salmon on top.
5. Serve with lemon wedges.

Nutritional Value

- Calories Approximately 400
- Protein 30g
- Healthy Fats 20g

Cooking Time 15 minutes

9. Lentil and Vegetable Stir-Fry

Ingredients
- 1 cup cooked lentils
- 1 cup mixed vegetables (bell peppers, broccoli, snap peas)
- 2 tablespoons soy sauce
- 1 tablespoon sesame oil
- 1 clove garlic, minced
- 1 teaspoon ginger, grated
- Green onions for garnish
- Sesame seeds for garnish

Preparation
1. In a wok or skillet, heat sesame oil.
2. Add minced garlic and grated ginger, sauté until fragrant.
3. Add mixed vegetables and stir-fry until crisp-tender.
4. Stir in cooked lentils and soy sauce, cook for an additional 2-3 minutes.
5. Garnish with green onions and sesame seeds.

Nutritional Value
- Calories Approximately 300
- Protein 15g
- Fiber 10g

Cooking Time 15 minutes

10. Baked Sweet Potato Fries

Ingredients

- 2 medium sweet potatoes, cut into fries
- 2 tablespoons olive oil
- 1 teaspoon paprika
- 1/2 teaspoon garlic powder
- Salt and pepper to taste

Preparation

1. Preheat the oven to 425°F (220°C) and line a baking sheet with parchment paper.
2. Toss sweet potato fries with olive oil, paprika, garlic powder, salt, and pepper in a bowl.
3. Spread the fries on the baking sheet in a single layer.
4. Bake for 20-25 minutes, turning halfway through, until crispy.

Nutritional Value

- Calories Approximately 200
- Fiber 6g
- Healthy Fats 8g

Cooking Time 25 minutes

DINNER RECIPES

Below are revised versions of the brain/mind diet recipes

1. Baked Salmon with Roasted Asparagus and Lemon-Dill Sauce

Ingredients
- 4 salmon fillets (6 ounces each)
- 1 bunch asparagus, trimmed
- 2 tablespoons olive oil
- Salt and pepper to taste
- Lemon-Dill Sauce
  - 1/4 cup Greek yogurt
  - 1 tablespoon freshly chopped dill
  - Zest and juice of 1 lemon

Preparation
1. Preheat the oven to 400°F (200°C).
2. Arrange salmon and asparagus on a baking sheet.
3. Drizzle with olive oil; season with salt and pepper.
4. Bake for 15-20 minutes until salmon is cooked.
5. Mix Greek yogurt, dill, lemon zest, and juice for the sauce.
6. Serve salmon and asparagus drizzled with Lemon-Dill Sauce.

Nutritional Value
- Calories Approx. 350
- Protein 30g

- Healthy Fats 20g

Cooking Time 20 minutes

2. Slow Cooker Chicken with Sweet Potato Mash

Ingredients
- 4 boneless, skinless chicken breasts
- 2 sweet potatoes, peeled and diced
- 1 cup chicken broth
- 2 cloves garlic, minced
- 1 teaspoon chopped rosemary
- Salt and pepper to taste
- 2 tablespoons olive oil

Preparation
1. Place chicken in the slow cooker.
2. Add sweet potatoes, chicken broth, garlic, rosemary, salt, and pepper.
3. Cook on low for 6-8 hours or high for 3-4 hours.
4. Mash sweet potatoes; serve with chicken.

Nutritional Value
- Calories Approx. 400
- Protein 35g
- Healthy Carbs 30g

Cooking Time 6-8 hours (slow cooker)

3. Grilled Lamb Chops with Sautéed Kale and Mushrooms

Ingredients
- 4 lamb chops
- 2 cups chopped kale
- 1 cup sliced mushrooms
- 2 tablespoons olive oil
- 2 cloves garlic, minced
- Salt and pepper to taste
- 1 teaspoon chopped thyme

Preparation
1. Preheat the grill to medium-high heat.
2. Season lamb chops with salt, pepper, and thyme.
3. Grill chops for 3-4 minutes per side.
4. Sauté kale and mushrooms with olive oil and garlic.
5. Serve lamb chops on sautéed kale and mushrooms.

Nutritional Value
- Calories Approx. 450
- Protein 35g
- Healthy Fats 25g

Cooking Time 10 minutes

4. Fish Tacos with Guacamole

Ingredients
- 1-pound white fish fillets (tilapia or cod)
- 8 small corn tortillas
- 1 cup shredded cabbage
- 1 cup halved cherry tomatoes
- 1/2 cup diced red onion
- 1/4 cup chopped cilantro
- Guacamole
  - 2 ripe avocados, mashed
  - Juice of 1 lime
  - Salt and pepper to taste

Preparation
1. Season fish fillets with salt and pepper.
2. Grill or pan-cook fish until flaky.
3. Warm tortillas; assemble tacos with fish, cabbage, tomatoes, onion, and cilantro.
4. Mix mashed avocados, lime juice, salt, and pepper for guacamole.
5. Serve tacos with a dollop of guacamole.

Nutritional Value
- Calories Approx. 400
- Protein 25g
- Healthy Fats 20g

Cooking Time 15 minutes

5. Vegetable Quinoa Bowl

Ingredients

- 1 cup cooked quinoa
- 1 cup broccoli florets
- 1 cup sliced bell peppers
- 1 cup halved cherry tomatoes
- 1 cup drained and rinsed chickpeas
- 2 tablespoons olive oil
- 1 teaspoon cumin
- Salt and pepper to taste
- Lemon wedges for serving

Preparation

1. Sauté broccoli, bell peppers, tomatoes, and chickpeas in olive oil.
2. Season with cumin, salt, and pepper.
3. Serve over cooked quinoa.
4. Garnish with lemon wedges.

Nutritional Value

- Calories Approx. 380
- Protein 15g
- Fiber 12g

Cooking Time 20 minutes

6. Grilled Vegetable and Hummus Wrap

Ingredients
- 1 whole-grain wrap
- 1 sliced zucchini
- 1 sliced eggplant
- 1 sliced red bell pepper
- 1/4 cup hummus
- 2 tablespoons crumbled feta cheese
- 1 tablespoon olive oil
- Salt and pepper to taste

Preparation
1. Grill zucchini, eggplant, and bell pepper slices with olive oil, salt, and pepper.
2. Spread hummus on the whole-grain wrap.
3. Layer grilled vegetables on the wrap.
4. Sprinkle with feta cheese.
5. Roll the wrap and secure with toothpicks if needed.

Nutritional Value
- Calories Approx. 350
- Protein 10g
- Healthy Fats 15g

Cooking Time 15 minutes

7. Slow Cooker Lentil Soup

Ingredients
- 1 cup dry green lentils
- 3 diced carrots
- 2 diced celery stalks
- 1 diced onion
- 3 cloves minced garlic
- 1 can (14 oz) diced tomatoes
- 6 cups vegetable broth
- 1 teaspoon cumin
- 1 teaspoon paprika
- Salt and pepper to taste
- Fresh parsley for garnish

Preparation
1. Rinse lentils and place in the slow cooker.
2. Add carrots, celery, onion, garlic, diced tomatoes, vegetable broth, cumin, paprika, salt, and pepper.
3. Cook on low for 8 hours or high for 4 hours.
4. Garnish with fresh parsley before serving.

Nutritional Value
- Calories Approx. 300
- Protein 15g
- Fiber 10g

Cooking Time 4-8 hours (slow cooker)

8. Eggplant Parmesan

Ingredients

- 2 large eggplants, sliced
- 2 cups marinara sauce
- 2 cups shredded mozzarella cheese
- 1 cup grated Parmesan cheese
- 1 cup breadcrumbs
- 2 beaten eggs
- 2 tablespoons olive oil
- Fresh basil for garnish

Preparation

1. Preheat the oven to 375°F (190°C).
2. Dip eggplant slices in beaten eggs, then coat with breadcrumbs.
3. Pan-fry eggplant in heated olive oil until golden.
4. Layer marinara sauce, eggplant, mozzarella, and Parmesan in a baking dish.
5. Repeat layers; bake for 25-30 minutes.
6. Garnish with fresh basil before serving.

Nutritional Value

- Calories Approx. 400
- Protein 20g
- Healthy Fats 15g

Cooking Time 30 minutes

9. Baked Tilapia with Spinach and Tomatoes

Ingredients
- 4 tilapia fillets
- 4 cups fresh spinach
- 2 cups halved cherry tomatoes
- 3 cloves minced garlic
- 1 sliced lemon
- 2 tablespoons olive oil
- Salt and pepper to taste

Preparation
1. Preheat the oven to 375°F (190°C).
2. Place tilapia fillets in a baking dish.
3. Surround with fresh spinach, cherry tomatoes, minced garlic, and lemon slices.
4. Drizzle with olive oil; season with salt and pepper.
5. Bake for 20-25 minutes until tilapia is cooked.

Nutritional Value
- Calories Approx. 320
- Protein 30g
- Healthy Fats 15g

Cooking Time 25 minutes

10. Mediterranean Pasta Salad

Ingredients
- 8 oz cooked whole-grain pasta
- 1 cup halved cherry tomatoes
- 1 diced cucumber
- 1/2 cup sliced Kalamata olives
- 1/4 cup finely chopped red onion
- 1/4 cup crumbled feta cheese
- Dressing
  - 3 tablespoons olive oil
  - 2 tablespoons balsamic vinegar
  - 1 teaspoon Dijon mustard
  - Salt and oregano to taste

Preparation
1. In a large bowl, combine cooked pasta, cherry tomatoes, cucumber, olives, red onion, and feta.
2. Whisk together olive oil, balsamic vinegar, Dijon mustard, salt, and oregano.
3. Pour the dressing over the pasta mixture; toss gently.

Nutritional Value
- Calories Approx. 350
- Protein 10g
- Healthy Fats 15g

Cooking Time 15 minutes

DESSERT RECIPES

Here are comprehensive explanations of the recipes tailored for brain health, covering ingredients, preparation methods, quantity details, nutritional values, and approximate cooking durations—all provided in US units.

1. Pumpkin Seed Energy Bites

Ingredients
- 1 cup of rolled oats
- 1/2 cup of pumpkin seeds
- 1/2 cup of nut butter (almond or peanut)
- 1/3 cup of honey or maple syrup
- 1/2 cup of dark chocolate chips
- 1 teaspoon of vanilla extract
- A pinch of salt

Preparation
1. In a food processor, blend rolled oats and pumpkin seeds until finely ground.
2. Add nut butter, honey or maple syrup, dark chocolate chips, vanilla extract, and a pinch of salt. Blend until well mixed.
3. Form the mixture into bite-sized balls and refrigerate for at least 30 minutes.

Nutritional Value
- Calories Approximately 150 per serving
- Protein 5g

- Healthy Fats 8g

Cooking Time 10 minutes

2. Blueberry Almond Oat Bars

Ingredients
- 2 cups of rolled oats
- 1 cup of almond flour
- 1/2 cup of melted coconut oil
- 1/3 cup of honey
- 1 teaspoon of vanilla extract
- 1 cup of fresh or frozen blueberries

Preparation
1. Preheat the oven to 350°F (175°C) and grease a baking dish.
2. Combine rolled oats, almond flour, melted coconut oil, honey, and vanilla extract in a bowl.
3. Press half of the mixture into the bottom of the prepared dish.
4. Sprinkle blueberries evenly over the crust.
5. Crumble the remaining oat mixture over the blueberries.
6. Bake for 25-30 minutes or until golden brown.

Nutritional Value
- Calories Approximately 200 per serving
- Protein 4g
- Healthy Fats 10g

Cooking Time 25-30 minutes

3. Walnut and Banana Bread

Ingredients
- 2 cups of mashed ripe bananas
- 1/2 cup of melted coconut oil
- 1/2 cup of honey
- 2 large eggs
- 1 teaspoon of vanilla extract
- 2 cups of all-purpose flour
- 1 teaspoon of baking soda
- 1/2 teaspoon of salt
- 1/2 cup of chopped walnuts

Preparation
1. Preheat the oven to 350°F (175°C) and grease a loaf pan.
2. In a large bowl, whisk together mashed bananas, melted coconut oil, honey, eggs, and vanilla extract.
3. In a separate bowl, combine flour, baking soda, and salt.
4. Add the dry ingredients to the banana mixture; stir until just combined.
5. Fold in chopped walnuts.
6. Pour the batter into the prepared loaf pan and bake for 60-65 minutes.

Nutritional Value
- Calories Approximately 250 per serving
- Protein 4g
- Healthy Fats 12g

Cooking Time 60-65 minutes

4. Turmeric Golden Milk Popsicles
Ingredients
- 2 cups of coconut milk
- 1 teaspoon of ground turmeric
- 1/2 teaspoon of ground ginger
- 1/4 cup of honey or maple syrup
- 1/2 teaspoon of vanilla extract
- A pinch of black pepper

Preparation
1. Warm coconut milk in a saucepan over medium heat.
2. Whisk in turmeric, ginger, honey or maple syrup, vanilla extract, and black pepper.
3. Allow the mixture to cool, then pour it into popsicle molds.
4. Freeze for at least 4 hours or until fully set.

Nutritional Value
- Calories Approximately 100 per popsicle
- Healthy Fats 6g

Cooking Time 10 minutes

5. Baked Apples with Walnuts and Cinnamon

Ingredients
- 4 large apples, cored and halved
- 1/2 cup of chopped walnuts
- 2 tablespoons of honey
- 1 teaspoon of ground cinnamon
- 1/4 teaspoon of nutmeg
- 1 tablespoon of melted butter (optional)

Preparation
1. Preheat the oven to 375°F (190°C) and grease a baking dish.
2. Place apple halves in the dish.
3. In a bowl, combine walnuts, honey, cinnamon, nutmeg, and melted butter.
4. Spoon the mixture onto each apple half.
5. Bake for 25-30 minutes or until apples are tender.

Nutritional Value
- Calories Approximately 150 per serving
- Protein 2g
- Healthy Fats 8g

Cooking Time 25-30 minutes

6. Berry Parfait

Ingredients

- 1 cup of Greek yogurt
- 1 cup of mixed berries (strawberries, blueberries, raspberries)
- 1/2 cup of granola
- 1 tablespoon of honey

Preparation

1. In a glass or bowl, layer Greek yogurt, mixed berries, and granola.
2. Repeat the layers.
3. Drizzle honey on top.

Nutritional Value

- Calories Approximately 300 per serving
- Protein 15g

Cooking Time 5 minutes

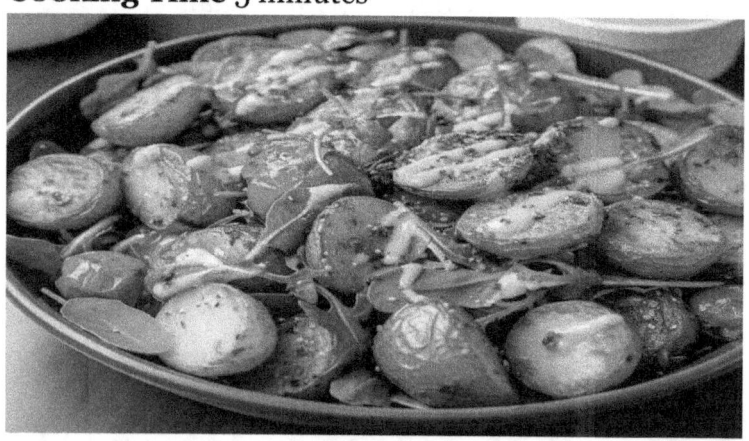

7. Dark Chocolate Avocado Mousse

Ingredients
- 2 ripe avocados
- 1/2 cup of unsweetened cocoa powder
- 1/2 cup of maple syrup
- 1 teaspoon of vanilla extract
- A pinch of salt
- Dark chocolate shavings for garnish

Preparation
1. In a food processor, blend avocados, cocoa powder, maple syrup, vanilla extract, and salt until smooth.
2. Refrigerate for at least 1 hour.
3. Serve topped with dark chocolate shavings.

Nutritional Value
- Calories Approximately 200 per serving
- Protein 3g
- Healthy Fats 12g

Cooking Time 10 minutes

_____
_____
_____
_____
_____
_____
_____

8. Chia Seed Pudding with Almond Butter

Ingredients
- 1/4 cup of chia seeds
- 1 cup of almond milk
- 1 tablespoon of almond butter
- 1 tablespoon of honey
- 1/2 teaspoon of vanilla extract
- Sliced almonds for topping

Preparation
1. In a bowl, whisk together chia seeds, almond milk, almond butter, honey, and vanilla extract.
2. Refrigerate for at least 4 hours or overnight.
3. Top with sliced almonds before serving.

Nutritional Value
- Calories Approximately 250 per serving
- Protein 7g
- Healthy Fats 15g

Cooking Time 4 hours

_____
_____
_____
_____
_____
_____
_____
_____

9. Coconut and Berry Smoothie Bowl

Ingredients
- 1 cup of mixed berries (strawberries, blueberries, raspberries)
- 1/2 banana
- 1/2 cup of coconut milk
- 1/4 cup of Greek yogurt
- 1 tablespoon of chia seeds
- 1 tablespoon of shredded coconut
- Granola for topping

Preparation
1. Blend mixed berries, banana, coconut milk, Greek yogurt, and chia seeds until smooth.
2. Pour into a bowl and top with shredded coconut and granola.

Nutritional Value
- Calories Approximately 280 per serving
- Protein 5g

Cooking Time 5 minutes

_____
_____
_____
_____
_____
_____

10. Yogurt and Mango Sorbet

Ingredients

- 2 cups of Greek yogurt
- 2 ripe mangoes, peeled and diced
- 1/4 cup of honey
- 1 tablespoon of lime juice
- Mint leaves for garnish

Preparation

1. In a blender, combine Greek yogurt, diced mangoes, honey, and lime juice.
2. Blend until smooth.
3. Pour the mixture into a shallow dish and freeze for 4 hours, stirring every hour.
4. Serve garnished with mint leaves.

Nutritional Value

- Calories Approximately 180 per serving
- Protein 10g

Cooking Time 4 hours

_____
_____
_____
_____
_____
_____
_____

SNACK AND SIDE RECIPES

Below are detailed explanations of the recipes for the brain/mind diet, encompassing ingredients, preparation techniques, quantity specifications, nutritional details, and anticipated cooking durations—all articulated in US units.

1. Avocado Toast with Crumbled Feta

Ingredients
- 2 slices of whole-grain bread
- 1 mashed ripe avocado
- 1/4 cup of crumbled feta cheese
- Salt and pepper to taste
- Optional Red pepper flakes for an extra kick

Preparation
1. Toast the whole-grain bread slices to your preference.
2. Evenly spread the mashed avocado over the toasted bread.
3. Sprinkle crumbled feta on top.
4. Season with salt, pepper, and, if desired, red pepper flakes.

Nutritional Value
- Calories Approximately 300
- Healthy Fats 15g
- Protein 10g

Cooking Time 5 minutes

2. Skinny Greek Yogurt Ranch Dip with Baby Carrots

Ingredients
- 1 cup of Greek yogurt
- 1 tablespoon dried dill
- 1 tablespoon dried parsley
- 1 teaspoon garlic powder
- 1 teaspoon onion powder
- 1 teaspoon dried chives
- Salt and pepper to taste
- Baby carrots for dipping

Preparation
1. Combine Greek yogurt, dried dill, dried parsley, garlic powder, onion powder, dried chives, salt, and pepper in a bowl.
2. Chill the dip in the refrigerator for at least 30 minutes.
3. Serve with baby carrots for a wholesome and crunchy snack.

Nutritional Value
- Calories Approximately 150 (for dip and carrots)
- Protein 15g
- Healthy Fats 5g

Cooking Time 5 minutes

3. Sweet Potato Fries with Honey Mustard Dip

Ingredients
- 2 sweet potatoes, cut into fries
- 2 tablespoons olive oil
- 1 teaspoon paprika
- 1 teaspoon garlic powder
- Salt and pepper to taste
- For the Honey Mustard Dip
  - 2 tablespoons Dijon mustard
  - 1 tablespoon honey

Preparation
1. Preheat the oven to 425°F (220°C).
2. Toss sweet potato fries with olive oil, paprika, garlic powder, salt, and pepper.
3. Spread the fries on a baking sheet and bake for 25-30 minutes.
4. Mix Dijon mustard and honey for the dip.
5. Serve sweet potato fries with the Honey Mustard Dip.

Nutritional Value
- Calories Approximately 250
- Fiber 6g
- Healthy Fats 8g

Cooking Time 30 minutes

4. Kale Chips with Parmesan

Ingredients

- 1 bunch kale, stems removed and torn into pieces
- 2 tablespoons olive oil
- 1/4 cup grated Parmesan cheese
- Salt and pepper to taste

Preparation

1. Preheat the oven to 300°F (150°C).
2. Toss kale pieces with olive oil, Parmesan, salt, and pepper.
3. Spread the kale on a baking sheet in a single layer.
4. Bake for 20-25 minutes until crisp.

Nutritional Value

- Calories Approximately 150
- Protein 8g
- Healthy Fats 10g

Cooking Time 25 minutes

_____
_____
_____
_____
_____
_____
_____
_____

5. Apple and Almond Butter Snack Wraps

Ingredients

- 2 whole-grain tortillas
- 2 tablespoons almond butter
- 1 apple, thinly sliced
- Cinnamon for sprinkling

Preparation

1. Spread almond butter evenly on each tortilla.
2. Place sliced apples on one side of the tortilla.
3. Sprinkle cinnamon over the apples.
4. Roll up the tortilla and slice into bite-sized wraps.

Nutritional Value

- Calories Approximately 300
- Protein 6g
- Healthy Fats 10g

Cooking Time 5 minutes

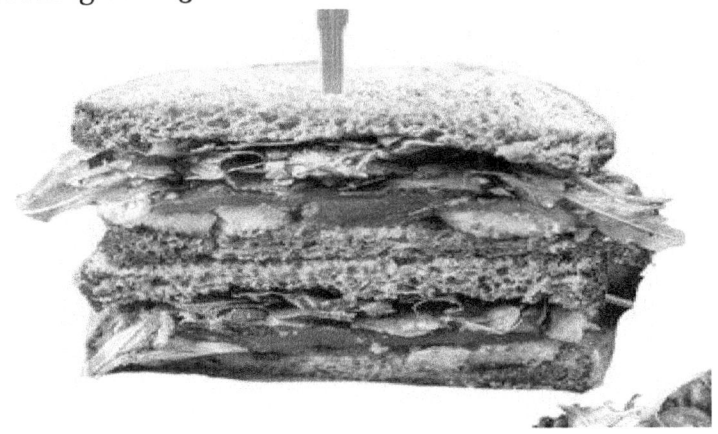

6. Broccoli and Cheese Bites

Ingredients
- 2 cups broccoli florets, steamed and chopped
- 1 cup cheddar cheese, shredded
- 1/2 cup breadcrumbs
- 2 eggs
- 1 teaspoon garlic powder
- Salt and pepper to taste

Preparation
1. Preheat the oven to 375°F (190°C) and grease a mini-muffin tin.
2. Combine chopped broccoli, cheddar cheese, breadcrumbs, eggs, garlic powder, salt, and pepper in a bowl.
3. Spoon the mixture into the mini-muffin tin.
4. Bake for 15-18 minutes until golden brown.

Nutritional Value
- Calories Approximately 200
- Protein 12g
- Healthy Fats 10g

Cooking Time 18 minutes

7. Zucchini Fritters with Greek Yogurt Sauce

Ingredients
- 2 medium zucchinis, grated and drained
- 1/2 cup breadcrumbs
- 1/4 cup grated Parmesan cheese
- 2 eggs
- 1 teaspoon dried oregano
- Salt and pepper to taste
- For the Greek Yogurt Sauce
  - 1/2 cup Greek yogurt
  - 1 tablespoon lemon juice
  - 1 teaspoon chopped fresh dill

Preparation
1. Combine grated and drained zucchini with breadcrumbs, Parmesan, eggs, oregano, salt, and pepper.
2. Form the mixture into fritters and cook in a skillet until golden brown on both sides.
3. For the sauce, mix Greek yogurt, lemon juice, and fresh dill.
4. Serve zucchini fritters with the Greek Yogurt Sauce.

Nutritional Value
- Calories Approximately 250
- Protein 15g
- Healthy Fats 8g

Cooking Time 15 minutes

8. Baked Parmesan Garlic Edamame

Ingredients
- 2 cups edamame, thawed if frozen
- 2 tablespoons olive oil
- 1/4 cup grated Parmesan cheese
- 2 cloves garlic, minced
- Salt and pepper to taste

Preparation
1. Preheat the oven to 375°F (190°C).
2. Toss edamame with olive oil, Parmesan, minced garlic, salt, and pepper.
3. Spread edamame on a baking sheet.
4. Bake for 15-20 minutes until crispy.

Nutritional Value
- Calories Approximately 220
- Protein 17g
- Healthy Fats 10g

Cooking Time 20 minutes

_____
_____
_____
_____
_____
_____

9. Cucumber Hummus Bites

Ingredients
- 1 cucumber, sliced into rounds
- 1/2 cup hummus
- Cherry tomatoes, halved
- Fresh basil leaves for garnish

Preparation
1. Top cucumber rounds with a small dollop of hummus.
2. Place a halved cherry tomato on each cucumber round.
3. Garnish with fresh basil leaves.

Nutritional Value
- Calories Approximately 150
- Protein 5g
- Healthy Fats 8g

Cooking Time 5 minutes

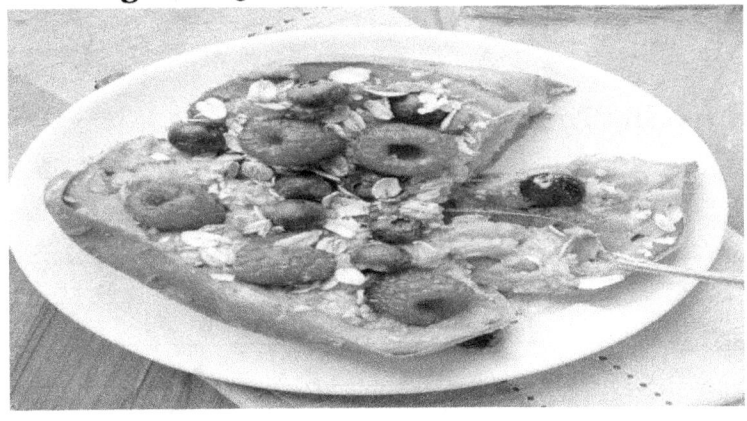

10. Roasted Chickpeas with Herbs and Spices

Ingredients
- 2 cans (15 oz each) chickpeas, drained and rinsed
- 2 tablespoons olive oil
- 1 teaspoon cumin
- 1 teaspoon paprika
- 1/2 teaspoon garlic powder
- Salt and cayenne pepper to taste

Preparation
1. Preheat the oven to 400°F (200°C).
2. Toss chickpeas with olive oil, cumin, paprika, garlic powder, salt, and cayenne pepper.
3. Spread chickpeas on a baking sheet.
4. Roast for 25-30 minutes until crispy.

Nutritional Value
- Calories Approximately 180
- Protein 8g
- Healthy Fats 5g

Cooking Time 30 minutes

_____
_____
_____
_____
_____
_____

SMOOTHIE RECIPES

Here are comprehensive explanations for the smoothie recipes tailored for brain/mind health, detailing ingredients, preparation steps, quantity measurements, nutritional values, and approximate blending times—all conveyed in US units.

1. Blueberry-Banana Smoothie

Ingredients
- 1 cup blueberries (fresh or frozen)
- 1 ripe banana
- 1/2 cup Greek yogurt
- 1/2 cup almond milk
- 1 tablespoon chia seeds
- Ice cubes (optional)

Preparation
1. Combine blueberries, banana, Greek yogurt, almond milk, and chia seeds in a blender.
2. Blend until a smooth consistency is achieved.
3. Optionally, add ice cubes and blend again.

Nutritional Value
- Calories Approximately 250
- Protein 8g
- Fiber 10g

Blending Time 2-3 minutes

2. Strawberry-Mango Smoothie

Ingredients
- 1 cup strawberries (fresh or frozen)
- 1/2 cup mango chunks (fresh or frozen)
- 1/2 cup plain yogurt
- 1/2 cup orange juice
- 1 tablespoon flaxseeds
- Ice cubes (optional)

Preparation
1. Combine strawberries, mango chunks, plain yogurt, orange juice, and flaxseeds in a blender.
2. Blend until a smooth consistency is achieved.
3. Optionally, add ice cubes and blend again.

Nutritional Value
- Calories Approximately 200
- Protein 6g
- Vitamin C 90mg

Blending Time 2-3 minutes

3. Banana-Oat Smoothie

Ingredients
- 2 ripe bananas
- 1/2 cup rolled oats
- 1 cup milk (dairy or plant-based)
- 1 tablespoon honey
- 1/2 teaspoon cinnamon
- Ice cubes (optional)

Preparation
1. Combine ripe bananas, rolled oats, milk, honey, and cinnamon in a blender.
2. Blend until a smooth consistency is achieved.
3. Optionally, add ice cubes and blend again.

Nutritional Value
- Calories Approximately 300
- Protein 8g
- Fiber 5g

Blending Time 2-3 minutes

_____
_____
_____
_____
_____
_____
_____
_____

4. Spinach-Mango Smoothie
Ingredients
- 2 cups fresh spinach leaves
- 1 cup mango chunks (fresh or frozen)
- 1/2 cup pineapple chunks
- 1/2 cup coconut water
- 1 tablespoon hemp seeds
- Ice cubes (optional)

Preparation
1. Combine fresh spinach leaves, mango chunks, pineapple chunks, coconut water, and hemp seeds in a blender.
2. Blend until a smooth consistency is achieved.
3. Optionally, add ice cubes and blend again.

Nutritional Value
- Calories Approximately 180
- Protein 5g
- Iron 3mg

Blending Time 2-3 minutes

_____
_____
_____
_____
_____
_____

5. Kale-Apple Smoothie

Ingredients
- 1 cup kale leaves, stems removed
- 1 apple, cored and chopped
- 1/2 cup green grapes
- 1/2 cup apple juice
- 1 tablespoon chia seeds
- Ice cubes (optional)

Preparation
1. Combine kale leaves, chopped apple, green grapes, apple juice, and chia seeds in a blender.
2. Blend until a smooth consistency is achieved.
3. Optionally, add ice cubes and blend again.

Nutritional Value
- Calories Approximately 160
- Protein 4g
- Vitamin K 547mcg

Blending Time 2-3 minutes

_____
_____
_____
_____
_____
_____
_____
_____

6. Avocado-Banana Smoothie

Ingredients
- 1/2 avocado, peeled and pitted
- 1 ripe banana
- 1/2 cup Greek yogurt
- 1/2 cup almond milk
- 1 tablespoon flaxseeds
- Ice cubes (optional)

Preparation
1. Combine avocado, ripe banana, Greek yogurt, almond milk, and flaxseeds in a blender.
2. Blend until a smooth consistency is achieved.
3. Optionally, add ice cubes and blend again.

Nutritional Value
- Calories Approximately 280
- Protein 7g
- Healthy Fats 15g

Blending Time 2-3 minutes

_____
_____
_____
_____
_____
_____
_____

7. Orange-Coconut Smoothie

Ingredients
- 2 oranges, peeled and segmented
- 1/2 cup coconut milk
- 1/2 cup plain yogurt
- 1 tablespoon coconut flakes
- 1 tablespoon honey
- Ice cubes (optional)

Preparation
1. Combine orange segments, coconut milk, plain yogurt, coconut flakes, and honey in a blender.
2. Blend until a smooth consistency is achieved.
3. Optionally, add ice cubes and blend again.

Nutritional Value
- Calories Approximately 220
- Protein 5g
- Vitamin C 90mg

Blending Time 2-3 minutes

_____

_____

_____

_____

_____

_____

_____

8. Pineapple-Carrot Smoothie

Ingredients

-1 cup pineapple chunks
- 1/2 cup carrot juice
- 1/2 cup Greek yogurt
- 1 tablespoon ginger, grated
- 1 tablespoon chia seeds
- Ice cubes (optional)

Preparation

1. Combine pineapple chunks, carrot juice, Greek yogurt, grated ginger, and chia seeds in a blender.
2. Blend until a smooth consistency is achieved.
3. Optionally, add ice cubes and blend again.

Nutritional Value

- Calories Approximately 200
- Protein 6g
- Vitamin A 6000 IU

Blending Time 2-3 minutes

_____
_____
_____
_____
_____
_____
_____

9. Peach-Coconut Smoothie

Ingredients
- 1 cup peaches, sliced (fresh or frozen)
- 1/2 cup coconut water
- 1/2 cup plain yogurt
- 1 tablespoon almond butter
- 1 tablespoon honey
- Ice cubes (optional)

Preparation
1. Combine sliced peaches, coconut water, plain yogurt, almond butter, and honey in a blender.
2. Blend until a smooth consistency is achieved.
3. Optionally, add ice cubes and blend again.

Nutritional Value
- Calories Approximately 230
- Protein 5g
- Healthy Fats 10g

Blending Time 2-3 minutes

_____
_____
_____
_____
_____
_____
_____
_____

10. Kiwi-Banana Smoothie

Ingredients
- 2 kiwis, peeled and sliced
- 1 ripe banana
- 1/2 cup almond milk
- 1/2 cup Greek yogurt
- 1 tablespoon honey
- Ice cubes (optional)

Preparation
1. Combine sliced kiwis, ripe banana, almond milk, Greek yogurt, and honey in a blender.
2. Blend until a smooth consistency is achieved.
3. Optionally, add ice cubes and blend again.

Nutritional Value
- Calories Approximately 190
- Protein 6g
- Vitamin C 120mg

Blending Time 2-3 minutes

_____
_____
_____
_____
_____
_____
_____

SOME STANDARD KITCHEN MEASUREMENTS AND THEIR EQUIVALENCE.

Here are some standard kitchen measurements and their corresponding values, essential for brain/mind diet recipes

1. Teaspoon (tsp)
   - Equal to 5 milliliters (ml)
   - Typically employed for modest quantities of spices, extracts, or fluid elements like honey.

2. Tablespoon (tbsp)
   - Equal to 15 milliliters (ml) or 3 teaspoons
   - Utilized for more substantial amounts of ingredients such as condiments, oils, or sauces.

3. Cup
   - Equal to 240 milliliters (ml)
   - A conventional measure for both dry and liquid components like flour, sugar, or milk.

4. Fluid Ounce (Fl oz)
   - Equal to 30 milliliters (ml)
   - Utilized for gauging liquids such as water, juice, or milk.

5. Pint
   - Equal to 16 fluid ounces or roughly 473 milliliters

- Commonly used for quantifying liquids in larger volumes.

6. Quart
- Equal to 32 fluid ounces or approximately 946 milliliters
- Frequently employed for more substantial liquid volumes in cooking or baking.

7. Gallon
- Equal to 128 fluid ounces or about 3,785 milliliters
- A larger unit applied for measuring bulk liquid volumes.

8. Ounce (oz)
- Equal to approximately 28.35 grams
- Utilized for measuring both dry and liquid ingredients, particularly in smaller amounts.

9. Pound (lb.)
- Equal to 16 ounces or roughly 453.592 grams
- Typically used for measuring larger quantities of ingredients like flour, sugar, or meat.

10. Gram (g)
- A metric unit of weight, frequently used for precision in measurements.
- Approximately 28.35 grams make up one ounce.

11. Milligram (mg)

- A smaller unit of weight, especially beneficial for measuring supplements or specific additives.
- One gram is equivalent to 1,000 milligrams.

These standardized kitchen measurements play a pivotal role in accurately executing brain/mind diet recipes, ensuring precise ingredient quantities for optimal nutritional outcomes.

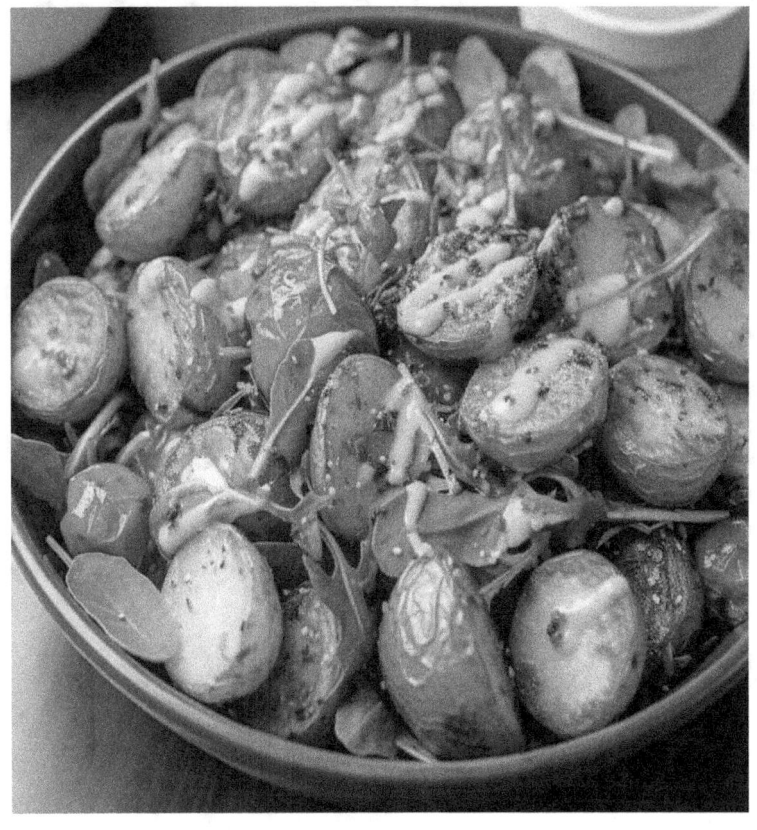

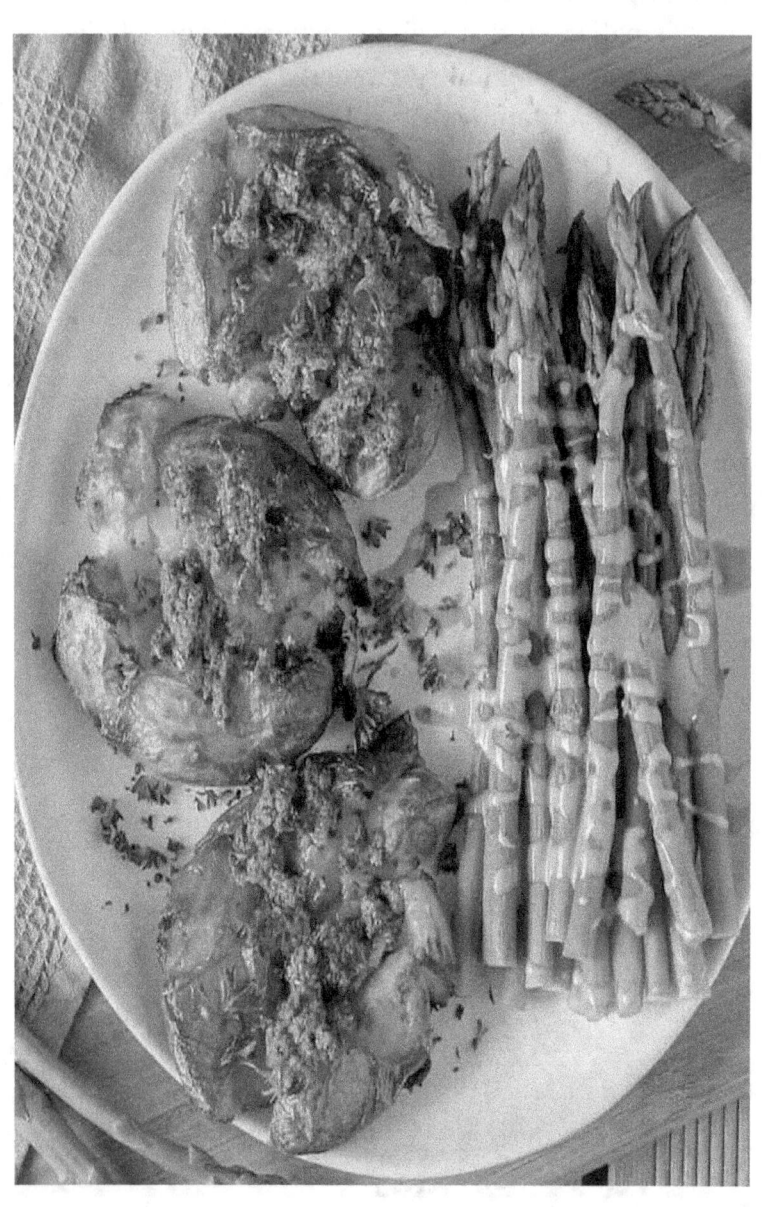

FOLLOW THE NEXT STEP

Moving beyond the Mind/Brain Diet unveils a captivating frontier in nutritional exploration and the enhancement of overall well-being. Let's delve into the subsequent echelon—the Next/Next Level of holistic health. This transcends the confines of individual dietary preferences, extending its reach to encompass a broader spectrum of lifestyle choices and mindfulness practices.

1. Tailored Nutritional Blueprints
- Crafting dietary plans customized to individual requisites, factoring in genetic makeup, metabolic intricacies, and personal health aspirations.
- Harnessing sophisticated technologies for meticulous nutrient monitoring and offering personalized meal recommendations.

2. Emphasis on the Gut-Brain Connection
- Acknowledging the intricate interplay between gut health and mental well-being.
- Infusing diets with probiotics, prebiotics, and fermented foods to cultivate a harmonious microbiome, with positive ramifications on cognitive functions.

3. Mindful Gastronomic Practices

- Wholeheartedly embracing mindfulness during meals, fostering a profound connection with the act of eating.
- Employing practices like intuitive eating and relishing each morsel to amplify satisfaction and optimize nutritional absorption.

4. Neurofeedback and Cognitive Augmentation

- Venturing into the realm of neurofeedback technologies to fine-tune brain functionality.
- Seamlessly integrating brain-training exercises and activities designed to enhance cognition into everyday routines.

5. Innovative Ingredients for Brain Enhancement

- Infusing cutting-edge ingredients, substantiated by scientific research, into dietary regimes—think adaptogens, nootropics, and functional mushrooms.
- Experimenting with nutrient-rich foods renowned for cognitive benefits, including turmeric, blueberries, and fatty fish.

6. Mindful Movement and Physical Activity

- Acknowledging the symbiotic relationship between physical exertion and mental well-being.

- Participating in mindful exercises such as yoga, tai chi, and aerobic activities as a holistic approach to overall well-being.

CONCLUSION

In Closing, embarking on the Next/Next Level of holistic well-being calls for an embrace of the concept that nurturing the mind transcends mere dietary choices. It necessitates a harmonious fusion of personalized nutrition, mindfulness rituals, and the infusion of cutting-edge scientific knowledge. By concurrently nurturing both our bodies and minds, we unlock the potential for a more vibrant, balanced, and satisfying life. Here's to the expedition of continual growth, where each conscious decision propels us further into the domain of heightened cognitive vitality and holistic wellness. Here's a toast to the Next/Next Level!

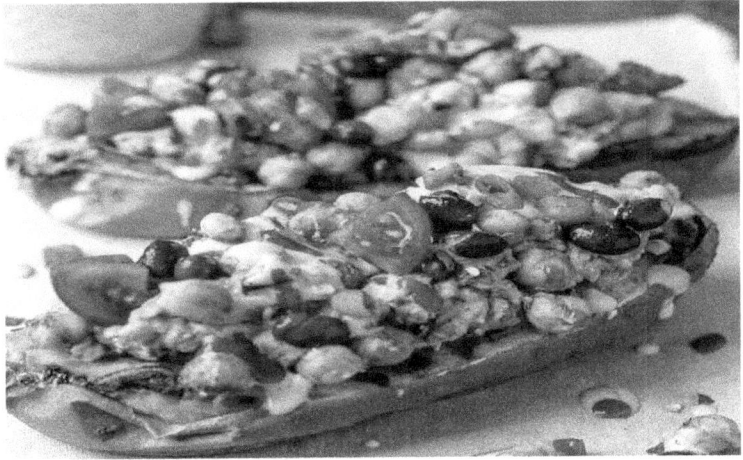

THANK YOU!!!

IF YOU FIND THIS BOOK TO BE INFORMATIVE, INSPIRING, OR SIMPLY ENJOYABLE, I WOULD BE IMMENSELY GRATEFUL IF YOU COULD SHARE YOUR THOUGHTS WITH OTHERS. YOUR HONEST REVIEW CAN MAKE A DIFFERENCE IN HELPING MORE INDIVIDUALS DISCOVER THE BENEFITS OF A NOURISHING AND MINDFUL APPROACH TO EATING. PLEASE CONSIDER LEAVING A REVIEW ON AMAZON AND SHARE YOUR EXPERIENCE.

THANK YOU ONCE AGAIN FOR CHOOSING THIS BOOK AS A COMPANION ON YOUR PATH TO A HEALTHIER, HAPPIER YOU.

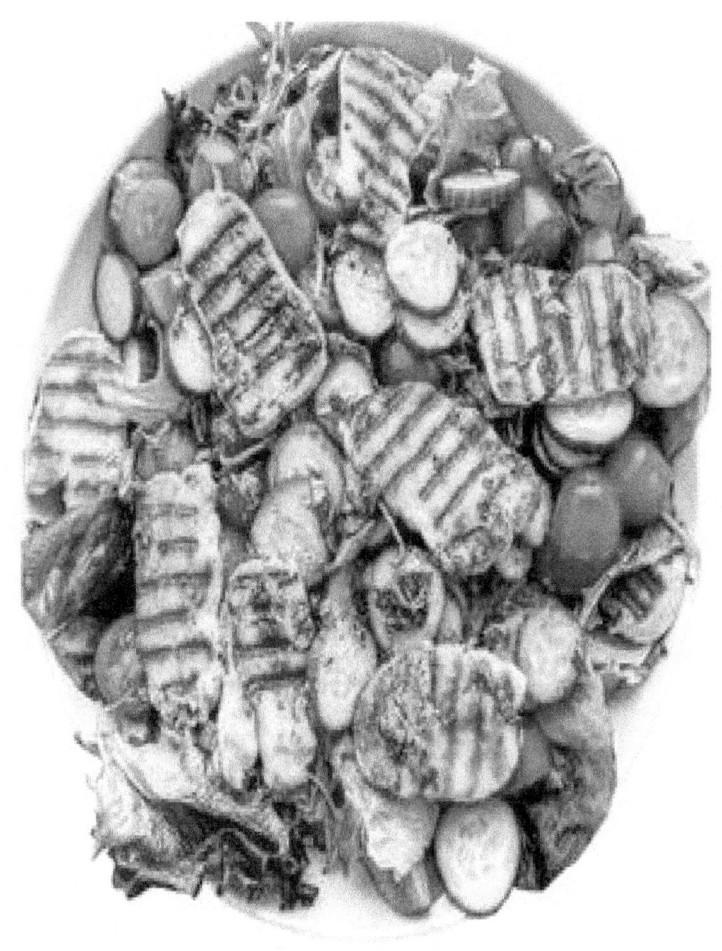

14 WEEKS RENAL DIET MEAL PLAN

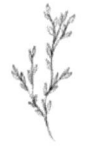 ## *Daily Meal Planner*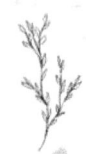

WEEK :   **MONTH :**   **YEAR :**

MONDAY	TUESDAY	WEDNESDAY

THURSDAY	FRIDAY	WEEKEND

NOTES

Daily Meal
Planner

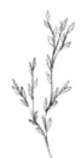
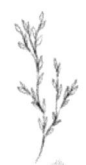

WEEK :　　　　MONTH :　　　　YEAR :

MONDAY	TUESDAY	WEDNESDAY

THURSDAY	FRIDAY	WEEKEND

NOTES

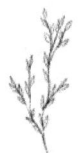

Daily Meal Planner

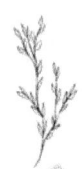

WEEK :   MONTH :   YEAR :

MONDAY	TUESDAY	WEDNESDAY

THURSDAY	FRIDAY	WEEKEND

NOTES

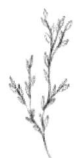 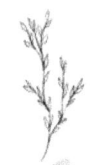

Daily Meal Planner

WEEK: MONTH: YEAR:

MONDAY

TUESDAY

WEDNESDAY

THURSDAY

FRIDAY

WEEKEND

NOTES

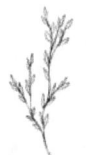

Daily Meal Planner

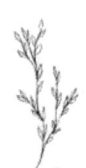

WEEK :　　　　MONTH :　　　　YEAR :

MONDAY	TUESDAY	WEDNESDAY

THURSDAY	FRIDAY	WEEKEND

NOTES

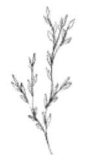

Daily Meal Planner

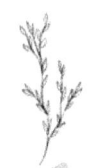

WEEK :   MONTH :   YEAR :

MONDAY	TUESDAY	WEDNESDAY

THURSDAY	FRIDAY	WEEKEND

NOTES

Daily Meal Planner

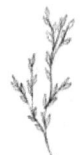
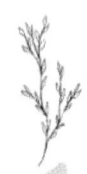

WEEK: **MONTH:**   **YEAR:**

MONDAY	TUESDAY	WEDNESDAY

THURSDAY	FRIDAY	WEEKEND

NOTES

Daily Meal Planner

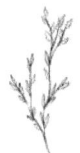
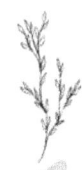

WEEK :   MONTH :   YEAR :

MONDAY	TUESDAY	WEDNESDAY

THURSDAY	FRIDAY	WEEKEND

NOTES

Daily Meal
Planner

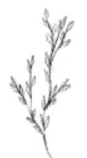
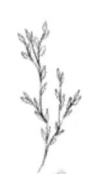

WEEK: **MONTH:**   **YEAR:**

MONDAY	**TUESDAY**	**WEDNESDAY**

THURSDAY	**FRIDAY**	**WEEKEND**

NOTES

Daily Meal Planner

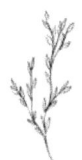 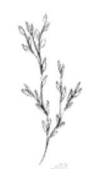

WEEK: **MONTH:** **YEAR:**

MONDAY	TUESDAY	WEDNESDAY

THURSDAY	FRIDAY	WEEKEND

NOTES

Daily Meal Planner

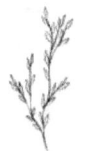 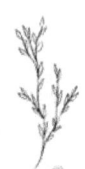

WEEK : **MONTH :** **YEAR :**

MONDAY	TUESDAY	WEDNESDAY

THURSDAY	FRIDAY	WEEKEND

NOTES

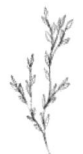

Daily Meal Planner

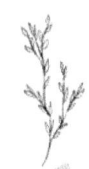

WEEK :   **MONTH :**   **YEAR :**

MONDAY	TUESDAY	WEDNESDAY

THURSDAY	FRIDAY	WEEKEND

NOTES

Daily Meal Planner

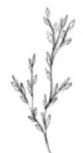
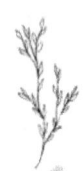

WEEK :   MONTH :   YEAR :

MONDAY	TUESDAY	WEDNESDAY

THURSDAY	FRIDAY	WEEKEND

NOTES

Daily Meal Planner

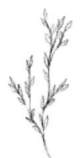 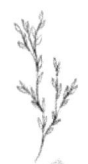

WEEK: _____   **MONTH:** _____   **YEAR:** _____

MONDAY	TUESDAY	WEDNESDAY

THURSDAY	FRIDAY	WEEKEND

NOTES

www.ingramcontent.com/pod-product-compliance
Lightning Source LLC
Chambersburg PA
CBHW071056290526
45795CB00004B/1525